Family health and medical guide:

"Family Health Essentials, A Beginner'sGuide to Recognizing Symptoms, Applying Remedies, and Exploring Natural and Herbal Medicine"
Bonus: 30 Day health guide

By
Florence J. Jacoby

Copyright

Disclaimer

Disclaimer: The information provided in this book, "Family Health and Medical Guide," is intended for general informational purposes only. It is not a substitute for professional medical advice, diagnosis, or treatment. Always seek the advice of your physician or qualified health provider with any questions you may have regarding a medical condition. The author and publisher do not endorse specific treatments or procedures mentioned in this guide, and they are not liable for any consequences resulting from the use of the information presented herein. Readers should use their discretion and consult healthcare professionals for personalized guidance based on individual circumstances.

BONUS: 30 Days health guide

Welcome to te Bonus: 30-Day Health Guide! This comprehensive guide is designed to kickstart your journey to a healthier lifestyle over the next month. Please note that individual results may vary, and it's crucial to consult with a healthcare professional before making significant changes to your diet or exercise routine.

Week 1: Establishing Foundations

Day 1-7: Setting Goals

- Define your health goals, whether it's weight loss, improved fitness, or overall well-being.

- Start a food journal to track your daily intake.

Week 2: Nutrition Makeover

Day 8-14: Healthy Eating Habits

- Focus on balanced meals with lean proteins, whole grains, fruits, and vegetables.

- Experiment with new recipes and cooking methods to make healthy eating enjoyable.

Week 3: Fitness Boost

Day 15-21: Get Moving

- Incorporate at least 30 minutes of moderate exercise daily.

- Try a mix of cardio, strength training, and flexibility exercises.

Week 4: Mind-Body Connection

Day 22-30: Stress Management and Mindfulness

- Practice relaxation techniques such as meditation or deep breathing.

- Prioritize sufficient sleep for overall well-being.

Bonus Tips:

1. Stay Hydrated: Aim for at least eight glasses of water daily.

2. Snack Smart: Choose nutrient-dense snacks like fruits, nuts, or yogurt.

3. Social Support: Share your journey with friends or family for motivation.

Remember, this 30-day guide is a starting point. Sustainable health is a lifelong journey, and it's essential to adapt these changes to fit your lifestyle. Listen to your body, make adjustments as needed, and celebrate your progress along the way. Here's to your health and well-being

Table of contents

10

Introduction

Welcome to "Family Health Essentials: A Beginner's Guide to Recognizing Symptoms, Applying Remedies, and Exploring Natural and Herbal Medicine." In this accessible journey into the realm of family well-being, we embark on a voyage of discovery—a guide crafted for beginners seeking a fundamental understanding of health. This book is more than just information; it's your companion in deciphering the language of your family's well-being. From understanding the basics of anatomy to discovering natural remedies, we'll navigate the seas of health together, ensuring that every member of your family can enjoy a healthier and happier life. So, let's begin this empowering journey toward a thriving and resilient family. As we embark on this enlightening journey, imagine a guide tailored not only to answer questions but to spark curiosity about the intricate dance of health within your family. In these pages, we'll unravel the mysteries of the human body, demystify symptoms, and empower you with simple, effective remedies. Beyond conventional wisdom, we'll delve into the world of natural and herbal medicine, offering gentle alternatives to nurture your family's well-being. This book is more than a resource; it's an invitation to take charge of your family's health narrative. Join us in this exploration, where knowledge meets empowerment, and each chapter unfolds a new chapter in your family's journey toward lasting vitality.

Brief explanation of the book's purpose

Imagine this book as your friendly guide on the journey to a healthier family. Its purpose? To make health simple and accessible for beginners. Whether it's understanding how your bodies work, recognizing when something's off, or finding easy remedies, this book has your back. We're not just sticking to the basics – we're exploring natural and herbal options, giving you gentle alternatives. So, if you want to empower your family with the know-how for a healthier, happier life, this guide is your trusted companion. Let's dive into a world where health is uncomplicated and within reach for everyone in your family.

Importance of family health for beginners

Understanding the significance of family health as beginners is like laying the essential groundwork for a life filled with joy and togetherness. It goes beyond merely preventing illnesses; it's about creating a foundation where every family member can thrive. Imagine fewer sick days and more quality time with loved ones, fewer trips to the doctor and more shared adventures. It's not just about health; it's about building stronger connections, nurturing a sense of well-being, and setting the stage for a future where everyone in the family can flourish. So, let's embark on this journey into family health together, unlocking the secrets to a vibrant and fulfilling life for you and your loved ones.

Chapter 1

Understanding Your Body

Alright, let's talk about getting to know your body it's like meeting a new friend. In this chapter, we are taking a bite approach to figure out how this amazing vessel of yours workshop. From the heart's metrical beat to the cooperation of your organs, we are keeping it easy and intriguing. No need for a medical degree; we are just unleashing the basics that help you make smart choices for your well-being. So, let's dive into this tone-discovery adventure. The more you get your body, the better you can treat it right and keep the good times rolling. Ready to be body musketeers? Let's roll! The mortal body is the entire structure of a mortal being. It's composed of numerous different types of cells that together produce atkins and latterly organs and also organ systems. They insure homeostasis and the viability of the mortalbody.Female(left wing) and manly(right) adult mortal bodies mugged in frontal(over) and rearward(below) perspectives. Naturally- being pubic, body, and facial hair has been designedly removed to show deconstruction. It comprises a head, hair, neck, torso(which includes the abdomen and tummy), arms and hands, legs and bases. The study of the mortal body includes deconstruction, physiology, histology and embryology. The body varies anatomically in given ways. Physiology focuses on the systems and organs of the mortal body and their functions. numerous systems and mechanisms interact in order to maintain homeostasis, with safe situations of substances similar as sugar and oxygen in the blood.The body is studied by health professionals, physiologists, anatomists, and artists to assist them in their work.

Simple overview of basic anatomy

Sure thing! Let's take a friendly perambulation through the basics of your body's design. Picture your body as a complex yet wonderfully systematized system. At its core is the heart, lifelessly pumping life through your modes. The lungs, your body's air cleansers, work alongside it, icing a constant force of oxygen. Your stomach and bowel, the digestive titlists, break down food to fuel your adventures. Bones give structure like a probative frame, while muscles power your every move. The brain, the ultimate command center, orchestrates it each, making opinions, storing recollections, and keeping the show handling. In this simple overview, we are not diving into the nitty- gritty; we are just getting acquainted with the major players. So, consider this your friendly preface to the inconceivable symphony that's your body! deconstruction is the identification and description of the structures of living effects. It's a branch of biology and drug. People who study deconstruction study the body, how it's made up, and how it works. The study of deconstruction dates back further than 2,000 yearsTrusted Source, to the Ancient Greeks. There are Three broad area— zootomy anatomy, human anatomy— phytotomy

Human anatomy

is the study of the structures of the mortal body. An understanding of deconstruction is crucial to the practice of drug and other areas ofhealth.The word " deconstruction " comes from the Greek words " corpus, " meaning " up, " and " book, " meaning " a slice. " Traditionally, studies of deconstruction have involved cutting up, or anatomizing, organisms. Now, still, imaging technology can show us important about how the inside of a body works, reducing the need for analysis. Below, learn about the two main approaches bitsy deconstruction and gross, or macroscopic, anatomy

Gross anatomy

In drug, gross, macro, or topographical deconstruction refers to the study of the natural structures that the eye can see. In other words, a person doesn't need a microscope to see these features. The study of gross deconstruction may involve analysis or noninvasive styles. The end is to collect data about the larger structures of organs and organ systems. In analysis, a scientist cuts open an organism — a factory or the body of a mortal or another beast — and examines what they discover outside.   Endoscopy is a tool for diagnosing illness, but it can also play a part in researchTrusted Source. It involves a scientist or fitting a long, thin tube with a camera at the end into different corridor of the body. By passing it through the mouth or rectum, for illustration, they can examine the inside of the gastrointestinal tract. There are also less invasive styles of disquisition. For illustration, to study the blood vessels of living creatures or humans, a scientist or may fit an opaque color, also use imaging technology, similar as angiography, to see the vessels that contain the color. This reveals how the circulatory system is working and whether there are any blockages. MRI reviews, CTreviews, PET reviews,X-rays, ultrasounds, and other types of imaging can also show what's passing inside a living body. Medical and dental scholars also perform analysis as part of their practical work during their studies. They may anatomize mortaL studies. They may dissect human corpses.

Human body systems

Students of gross anatomy learn about the major systems of the body.
There are 11 organ systems in the human body:
the skeletal system
the muscular system
the lymphatic system

the respiratory system
the digestive system
the nervous system, including the central and autonomic systems
the endocrine system, which regulates hormone production
the cardiovascular system, including the heart
the urinary system
the reproductive system
the integumentary system, which includes the skin, hair, and nails, among other areas

Chapter 2

Building Healthy Habits

We all know that eating well can extend our lives and improve our overall well-being. Perhaps you've already made an effort to improve your diet, increase your exercise or sleep, give up smoking, or manage your stress. It's not simple. However, studies reveal ways to improve your capacity to establish and maintain a healthy lifestyle.

NIH behavior change specialist Dr. Susan Czajkowski says, "It's frustrating to experience setbacks when you're trying to make healthy changes and reach a goal." "The good news is that there are tried-and-true methods you can employ to position yourself for success, as demonstrated by decades of research."

Numerous actions you do both now and in the future have an impact on your health and quality of life. By making healthy decisions, you can lower your risk for the most prevalent, expensive, and avoidable health issues, such obesity, type 2 diabetes, cancer, heart disease, and stroke.

Recognize Your Patterns

Daily routines, such as brushing your teeth or having a few drinks at night, can develop into habits. Repetitive positive activities might alter your brain in ways that may make it difficult to break bad habits. Habits frequently become habitual and occur without conscious awareness.

"Behavior change begins with raising awareness of your regular activities," says Dr. Lisa Marsch, a behavior change specialist at Dartmouth College. "Observe your behavior patterns and the things that lead to the unhealthy habits you wish to break."

Perhaps you overindulge in food while watching TV, or you go out with friends to smoke during breaks even though you don't want to. According to Marsch, "you can figure out how to break those patterns and make new ones." For example, eat meals without watching TV or go for walks with friends or other healthful activities.

Create a Strategy

Create a plan that outlines the precise steps you'll take to achieve your modest, realistic goals.

Try taking a different route to avoid buying junk food from the vending machine at work every day, and pack nutritious snacks from home instead, advises Czajkowski.

"Whenever feasible, choose the healthy option when it's easier."

Think about the things you believe you'll need to succeed. How can you alter your surroundings to help you achieve your objectives? It may be necessary for you to find a special place to unwind, clear out temptations, or stock up on nutritious foods.

Involve your loved ones and friends. According to research, people often adopt the same health-related habits as their friends and family. Bring them along, offer them encouragement, and assist you in staying on course.

It's also critical to prepare for setbacks. Consider what could thwart your greatest intentions to have a healthier lifestyle. How can you resist the urge to revert to old habits or make unhealthy decisions when faced with unforeseen circumstances or difficult times?

Remain on Course

Making healthy changes for yourself may be gratifying and thrilling. However, there will also be moments when you question your ability to persevere.

Marsch suggests, "Identify negative thoughts and replace them with realistic, productive ones."

Record-keeping can be useful. You can record details about your food, exercise routine, stress levels, and sleep habits using a paper journal, computer application, or smartphone app. People who maintained their weight loss for a year or more after losing at least thirty pounds were found to have constantly monitored their progress.

Czajkowski advises holding on "even when you think you're about to fall off the wagon."

"Keep an eye on your actions. You can sometimes learn the most when you feel like you're failing.

Digital solutions, such as mobile apps, that could help you in a time of need are being developed by Marsch and others. In order to improve our capacity to measure, monitor, and regulate our behavior, her team is also utilizing technology.

"The more self-control you exercise, the more proficient you get at it," asserts Dr. Leonard Epstein, a behavior modification and decision-making expert at the University at Buffalo. "You become capable of acting and responding in different ways."

Consider the Future

According to Epstein's research, some people find it more difficult than others to control their impulses. He refers to this as "delay discounting," in which the bigger advantages of delaying are discounted in favor of less substantial instant gains. This may result in unsafe sexual activity, substance addiction, binge drinking, excessive shopping, or overeating.

"Episodic future thinking, or vividly imagining future positive experiences or rewards, can teach you to postpone immediate gratification," he says. It's a fantastic approach to improve your capacity to decide what's best for you in the long term. Epstein is currently researching ways to help those who are at risk of type 2 diabetes avoid developing the condition.

It can be beneficial to consider how a change could improve your life and help your body heal. Within a day of quitting smoking, your chance of having a heart attack decreases. Improved relationships can result from stress reduction. Making even modest dietary and exercise changes can lower your risk of disease and increase your life expectancy.

Have patience.

Occasionally, attempting to adopt healthy habits may be impeded by other health concerns.

"If you're having a lot of trouble with these habits, consider whether there may be more going on," Czajkowski advises. "Unhealthy behaviors, for instance, can be linked to mental health conditions like depression and anxiety."

You're never too old, too fat, or too out of shape to make healthy changes. A health expert can work with you to address any underlying issues to make change feel easier and help you be more successful. Try out several tactics until you determine which one suits you the most.

It's acceptable if things don't go according to plan, according to Czajkowski. "A process is change. The most crucial thing is to keep going forward.

Make Sensible Decisions

Establish Healthful Habits

Organize. Determine harmful tendencies and stressors. Make sensible objectives. Steps to assist you reach them should be written down.

Modify your environment. Look for simple strategies to choose healthier options. Take temptations away. Strive to make improvements in your neighborhood, such as secure walkways.

Request assistance. Seek out the support of friends, family, neighbors, coworkers, or organizations, or invite them to join you.

Take up a lot of healthful hobbies with your time. Try engaging in your favorite pastime, exercising, or hanging out with loved ones.

Monitor your development. Keep track of your progress to ensure that you don't make the same mistakes twice.

Think ahead to the future. To continue on course, consider the benefits in the future.

Give yourself a reward. When you reach a minor objective or milestone, treat yourself to something beneficial, like a massage or some alone time.

Have patience. It takes time to improve, and obstacles arise. Prioritize progress over perfection.

Chapter 3

Preventing Common Illness

- Allergies
- .Colds and flu
- Diarrhea
- Headaches
- Mononucleosis

- Stomach Aches

Allergies

Allergies are an immune response triggered by allergens, an ordinarily harmful substance.

Causes

People with allergies have especially sensitive immune systems that react when they contact allergens.

Common allergens include:

- foods (nuts, eggs, milk, soy, shellfish, wheat)
- pollen
- mold
- latex
- pet dander

Symptoms

Because there are so many possible causes, the symptoms of allergies vary widely. Airborne allergens, like pollen and pet dander, are likely to cause:

- Eye irritation
- Runny nose
- Stuffy nose
- Puffy, watery eyes
- Sneezing
- Inflamed, itchy nose and throat

Allergens that are consumed, like foods or certain medications, can cause:

- Hives or skin rashes

- Gastrointestinal distress (diarrhea, nausea, vomiting, excessing gas, indigestion)
- Tingling or swelling of the lips, face, or tongue
- Itchiness
- Difficulty breathing or wheezing
- Fainting/ or lightheadedness

In cases of a more extreme response, called anaphylaxis, symptoms are severe and life-threatening.

Treatment

The easiest and most effective way to treat allergies is to get rid of or avoid the cause. Where unavoidable, some lifestyle changes can reduce your allergy symptoms. For example, if you are allergic to dust mites, make an effort to keep your room clean and free of dust by frequent vacuuming, dusting, and washing of bedding.

For pollen allergies, avoid being outside when pollen counts are high and keep the windows to your room shut.

Because it is very difficult to avoid certain allergens, medication may be necessary to lessen symptoms caused by allergens, other than food and drugs.

- **Antihistamines**: help relieve or prevent the sneezing, itchy eyes and throat, and postnasal drip that the allergen may cause. They are sold in many forms (i.e., pills, nasal sprays, liquids, etc.).

- **Decongestants:** help reduce congestion in your nasal membranes by narrowing the blood vessels that supply those membranes. They can be purchased in several forms (liquid, pill or nasal spray) and may be used with an antihistamine or alone to treat nasal swelling related to allergies. Limit use of nasal sprays to fewer than two to three days in a row because prolonged use can cause the nasal membrane swells, resulting in severe nasal obstruction.

- **Anti-inflammatory agents (e.g., corticosteroid):** help reduce swelling of the airways, nasal congestion and sneezing. Typically taken as a nasal spray. Some people report that corticosteroids irritate nasal passages.
- **Allergy shots:** recommended for serious allergy sufferers, this series of shots are administered by a healthcare provider and contain small amounts of the allergens that cause you discomfort. The goal of allergy shots is to enable your immune system to build better defenses against allergens.

Some allergies go away with age, but others are lifelong.

Prevention

- Avoid the outdoors between 5-10 a.m. and save outside activities for late afternoon or after a heavy rain, when pollen levels are lower.
- Keep windows in your living spaces closed to lower exposure to pollen.
- To keep cool, use air conditioners and avoid using window and attic fans.
- Wear a medical alert bracelet or other means to communicate to others about your allergy in case of a reaction.

- Discuss a prescription for epinephrine (e.g., EpiPen) with your healthcare provider, if you have risk of serious allergic reaction.
- Review product labels carefully before buying or consuming any item
- Know what you are eating or drinking.

Colds and flu

Colds and influenza (flu) are the most common illnesses among college students.

Causes

Both of these illnesses are upper respiratory infections, meaning they involve your nose, throat, and lungs. Viruses cause both colds and flu by increasing inflammation of the membranes in the nose and throat.

Most transmission of these viruses occurs via hand-to-hand contact.

Symptoms

Flu symptoms come on suddenly and affect the body all over. Flu symptoms are usually more serious than a cold and include:

- fever (100° F),
- headache,
- more intense pain and fatigue, and
- more severe, often dry cough.

When you get the flu, you are also more prone to bronchitis, sinus, and ear infections.

Cold symptoms mostly affect above the neck and include:

- a runny or stuffy nose (nasal congestion),
- sneezing,
- sore throat, and
- cough.

You may also experience a mild headache, body aches or a low grade fever. Typically, a cold lasts 2-14 days.

Treatment

If any problem is causing you discomfort, you should seek medical care.

Seek medical attention promptly if you have:

- a fever of 102° F or greater (which may indicate a more serious infection),
- a persisting cough, especially with a significant fever (which could indicate pneumonia),
- a persistent sore throat (especially if runny nose does not develop - which could indicate a strep infection), or
- any cold lasting more than 10 days.

Because colds and flu are caused by viruses, they cannot be cured by antibiotics. There are tips to help you feel better and strengthen your immune system to fight illness:

- Rest more than usual and avoid exercise until symptoms are gone.

- Drink lots of clear fluids (e.g., water, tea).
- Stay away from cigarette smoke.
- Do not take antibiotics unless specifically prescribed for you to cure the illness from which you currently suffer.
- Avoid drinking alcohol because it weakens your immune system and may interact with medications.
- Avoid caffeine, which can increase congestion and dehydration.
- Eat a well-balanced diet, including fruits, vegetables, and grains.

More Specific Remedies for Comfort

RUNNY NOSE/CONGESTION:

- Decongestants (e.g. pseudoephedrine) can relieve a runny nose and congestion, but these medications can inhibit sleep and suppress appetite.
- Salt water nasal sprays (e.g. NaSal or Ocean) can ease nasal congestion and thin mucus. However, excessive use of medicated nose sprays, like Afrin, can cause dependence and may make congestion worse.
- Humidifiers and hot showers can help to moisten nasal passages and clear mucus.

COUGH:

- Dextromethorphan is an effective cough suppressant, but because a cough is a protective reflex, it is not usually a bad thing. Take dextromethorphan if your cough is interfering with sleep or work.
- Water vapor from humidifiers and showers can help loosen the mucus causing a cough, as can chicken soup.

SORE THROAT:

- Phenol in lozenges and sprays is an effective pain reliever for sore throats.
- Gargling with warm saltwater (1 tsp. salt in one cup of warm water) every four hours may help ease pain by reducing swollen tonsils.

- Drinking tea with lemon (with or without honey).

FEVER/PAIN:

- Acetaminophen, Aspirin, Ibuprofen. If symptoms are severe, you may alternate acetaminophen and ibuprofen every two hours for pain or fever relief.

Prevention

UHS offers flu shots to Princeton students at a reduced cost every fall. Even though getting a flu shot will not completely eliminate your chances of developing the flu, it will certainly reduce the risk. Each year, a new vaccine made from inactivated (killed) influenza viruses is formulated. Since it may take the immune system time to respond to the vaccination, the inactivated vaccine should be given 6 to 8 weeks before flu season begins in order to prevent infection or reduce the severity of the illness.

The flu is probably only contagious during the first three days of illness, and the incubation period is 24-72 hours, meaning you might not show symptoms for three days after contracting the virus. It is rare to catch a cold virus through the air – most transmission occurs via hand-to-hand contact. To prevent colds, flu, and other illnesses, follow these tips:

- Wash your hands often (which is good advice for keeping healthy in any situation). Keep them away from your nose, eyes, and mouth. Use an instant hand sanitizer when you can't wash your hands.
- Get regular exercise and eat well.
- Follow good sleep habits.
- Get a flu shot each fall (offered to all students at a lower cost by UHS each fall)

Conjunctivitis ("pink eye")

Causes

Conjunctivitis, an inflammation of the transparent membrane (conjunctiva) that lines your eyelids and part of your eyeballs, has several possible causes. It could be a bacterial or viral infection, an allergic reaction to pollen or animal dander, or a result of chemical irritants (smoke, chlorine, lens solution, etc.).

Symptoms

These symptoms may last a few hours to several weeks: redness, itching, tearing, burning sensation, pus-like discharge and/or crusting of the eyelids. Because conjunctivitis causes inflammation of the small blood vessels in the conjunctiva to become more prominent, the whites of your eyes will appear pink or red. When you wake you are likely to feel that your eyelids are pasted shut, and your vision may not be as clear as usual.

Treatment

Because pink eye is highly contagious, early diagnosis is important. Bacterial cases can be cured with antibiotic eye drops, viral conjunctivitis clears up on its own, and allergic reactions can be treated with various types of eye drops. Here are some general tips:

- Wash your hands frequently to prevent spreading an existing infection to your other eye, and to other people.

- Don't rub your eyes.
- Use a cool wet washcloth to soak off any crusting.
- Use a warm or cool compress to reduce discomfort.
- Discard eye make-up because it may cause future infection.
- Wash any clothing that may be contaminated, including towels and pillowcases. Try to use clean towels and pillowcases everyday.
- Avoid wearing contact lenses and discard current lenses.
- If eye drops are prescribed, place drop in pocket formed by pulling down lower

lid. Make sure you don't touch the bottle to the eye in order to prevent contamination.

- If the infection does not improve in 2 or 3 days, make an appointment for re-evaluation.

Prevention

Pink eye is extremely contagious, so if you know someone who is infected, make sure you do not expose yourself to contact with the person's eye fluid. The infection can easily be passed via keyboards, doorknobs, make-up, pens, gym equipment, and a vast number of other items. To protect yourself, wash your hands frequently, avoid touching your eyes, and wash anything that may be contaminated.

Diarrhea

Causes

- Bacterial infection, caused by contaminated food or water
- Viral infection
- Parasites, which can enter the body through food or water
- Food intolerance, such as the inability to digest lactose, the sugar in milk
- Overuse of alcohol or laxatives
- Medication, such as some antibiotics or antacids containing magnesium
- Menstrual cramps

- Stress or a panic attack

Symptoms

- watery, loose stools
- frequent bowel movements
- cramping or pain in the abdomen, nausea, bloating
- possibly fever or bloody stools, depending on the cause

Treatment

Usually diarrhea will clear up on its own in a day or two, but a prolonged case may cause complications. The most important concern is dehydration. If you have symptoms of dehydration, a fever above 102° F, bloody stools (black and tarry), severe abdomen or rectum pain, or diarrhea lasting more than 3 days you should consult a physician. Here's some advice for taking care of diarrhea yourself:

- Avoid foods that are milk-based, greasy, high-fiber, or very sweet because these are likely to aggravate diarrhea.
- Avoid caffeine and alcohol.
- Do not eat solid food if you have signs of dehydration (thirst, light-headed, dark urine). Instead, drink about 2 cups of clear fluids per hour (if vomiting isn't present), such as sports drinks and broth. Water alone is not enough because your

body needs sodium and sugar to replace what it's losing.

- Avoid high sugar drinks, like apple juice, grape juice, and soda, which can pull water into the intestine and make the diarrhea persist.
- Don't drink clear liquids exclusively for more than 24 hours.
- Begin eating normal meals within 12 hours, but stick to food that is bland and won't irritate your intestine. Some doctors suggest the "BRAT" diet which includes foods that are low in fiber, fat, and sugar. BRAT stands for Bananas, Rice, Applesauce, and Toast.

- Use over-the-counter lactobacillus acidophilus capsules or tablets. These bacteria help maintain a healthy intestine, and are found in yogurt with live active cultures.
- Decrease level of exercise until symptoms are gone.
- Over-the-counter drugs, such as Imodium A-D, should only be used if absolutely necessary because it is important to let diarrhea flush out the bacteria or parasite that's causing the infection.

Headaches

Everyone suffers the occasional mild headache, but if you experience debilitating pain and/or abnormally frequent headaches, you probably want to find relief. There are countless causes of headaches, which differ for each person, so you'll have to do some experimenting to figure out the cause of your pain. Fortunately, the vast majority of headaches are primary headaches, not the result of underlying medical conditions. The three most common types are cluster, tension-type, and migraine.

A cluster headache affects a specific point of the head, often the eye, and is characterized by sharp, piercing pain. Migraine and tension-type headaches are far more common. "Tension" headaches are now called "tension-type" headaches because pain is not only caused by stress, but also poor posture, depression, and even sexual activity. In fact, recent studies have shown a connection between low serotonin levels and so-called "tension" headaches.

Causes

The cause of a headache is often elusive. Although it may seem that your head is pounding for no reason, there is always an explanation for pain. To find out the cause of your headaches, keep a log. Write down the date and time each headache starts and stops, the location of the pain, the nature and severity of the pain, and any factors that seem to trigger the headaches (food, stress, menstrual cycle, medicine, etc.).

Some of the many causes of headaches:

- Emotional and physical stress
- Fatigue
- Irregular sleep habits (sleeping too much or too little)
- Skipping meals
- Caffeine use or withdrawal
- Hormonal factors, such as menstruation
- Monosodium glutamate (MSG)
- Foods with nitrates, such as hot dogs
- Alcohol

- Some medicines
- Certain foods, including red wine, chocolate, aged cheeses, pickled foods, nuts, and aspartame
- Changes in weather, altitude, or time zone

Symptoms

Just as the causes vary for each headache sufferer, so do the symptoms and severity of pain. Health professionals can often diagnose the type of headache you suffer based on your symptoms.

Symptoms of a migraine:

- pulsing or throbbing quality

- begins with intense pain on one side of the head, which eventually spreads
- felt on one or both sides of the head
- lasts several hours
- severe enough to interfere with routine activities
- may be accompanied by nausea or vomiting
- Sometimes preceded by visual changes, such as an aura of zigzag lines or flashes of light
- light and noise can make the headache worse, while sleep tends to relieve symptoms

Symptoms of a tension-type headache:

- constant, dull ache
- felt on both sides of the head
- a feeling of squeezing or pressure
- does not usually interfere with routine activities
- lasts from 30 minutes to a few days

Treatment

- Ice pack held over the eyes or forehead
- Heating pad set on low or hot shower to relax tense neck and shoulder muscles
- Sleep, or at least resting in a dark room
- Taking breaks from stressful situations
- Regular exercise to increase endorphin levels and relax muscles. Even if you already have a headache, exercising may

relieve the pain. However, intense exercise may bring on a headache.

- Occasional use of over-the-counter medicines such as acetaminophen, ibuprofen, or aspirin can relieve both migraine and tension headaches. *
- Prescription drugs for severe headaches

* Overuse of pain medicine can actually result in more frequent headaches. Most pain-relieving medicines used to treat headaches can cause "analgesic rebound headaches" if used too often.

Prevention

- Be aware of early symptoms so you can try to stop the headache as soon as it begins.
- Don't smoke, and if you do, quit.
- Don't skip meals.
- Cut down on caffeine and alcohol (reduce caffeine intake gradually because withdrawal may cause headaches).
- Stop all over-the-counter medicines and herbal remedies.
- Maintain a regular eating and sleeping schedule.
- Exercise regularly.

- Incorporate relaxation activities into your daily routine, such as meditation, yoga, stretching exercises, and massage
- Improve your posture, possibly by adjusting your workstation.

Chapter 4

Quick Fixes for Everyday Ailments

Aches, pains, and mild discomforts are an inevitable part of daily life in all its busyness. This chapter is your go-to resource for quick fixes to common illnesses that could throw off the household routine temporarily. Let's look at doable solutions for typical problems so you can take them on head-on.

1. Tension and Headaches: * Treatment: Drinking plenty of water and practicing

relaxation techniques; * Reason: Stress and dehydration are common causes of headaches. Drink plenty of water and use relaxation methods to release stress, such deep breathing or light stretching.

2. Distressed Stomach: * Cure: Ginger tea or peppermint tea; * Justification: Both ginger and peppermint are well-known for their digestive qualities. Drinking tea with peppermint leaves or other ginger-infused drinks might help soothe nausea and upset stomachs.

3. Small Cuts and Scrapes: * Treatment: Wash with a gentle soap and water, then cover with a bandage and antiseptic

ointment. * Justification: It's important to keep small wounds clean to avoid infection. After giving the region a quick wash with mild soap and water, bandage it to provide protection and apply an antibacterial ointment.

4. Sore Muscles: * Treatment: Warm compress and light stretching * Justification: Warm compresses help ease sore muscles, and light stretching increases range of motion and lessens pain. Use these treatments to relieve your regular muscle aches.

5. Common Cold: * Treatment: Drink plenty of water, get plenty of rest, and eat

warm soups. * Interpretation: It is important to drink plenty of water, get plenty of rest, and eat warm soups to combat a common cold. These techniques can aid in symptom relief and hasten healing.

6. Insomnia or restlessness: * Solutions include creating a nightly schedule, avoiding electronics before bed, and practicing relaxation methods.

* Explanation: Establishing a regular bedtime routine, avoiding electronics before bed, and engaging in relaxation exercises all improve the quality of sleep and help with restlessness or insomnia.

7. Allergies: * Treatment: Recognizing triggers, taking over-the-counter antihistamines, and maintaining allergen-free living environments Explanation: To reduce discomfort, managing allergies entails recognizing triggers, using antihistamines as needed, and keeping allergen-free settings at home. 8. Tension headaches: * Treatment: Shoulder and neck stretches, warm compress, and mindfulness exercises

Chapter 5

Nurturing Mental Wellness

Although self-care techniques have their advantages, there can be occasions when more assistance is required. It is critical to understand that consulting mental health professionals is a legitimate and brave step on the road to recovery and development. Black community mental health resources, like culturally competent therapists and counselors, offer specialized care that recognizes the particular difficulties that members of the community confront. When it comes to resolving mental health issues and promoting personal development, having access to these resources can be revolutionary.

Developing Resilience: Finding Strength in Difficulties

Being resilient is a crucial quality that enables people to overcome obstacles in life and recover from failures. Resilience has long been seen in the Black community as a pillar of strength that has helped generations of people persevere despite hardship.

Recognizing the power of our current actions while simultaneously appreciating the strength of our ancestors is essential to building resilience. Accepting our resilient past might encourage us to take on the problems of the present with a sense of resolve and optimism.

Community Assistance: Encouraging One Another

In the Black community, mental wellness is greatly enhanced by communal support. Establishing a network of caring that empowers and uplifts its members can be achieved by coming together to help one another via common experiences and wisdom.

Support groups and community-based organizations can be important assets for mental wellness programs because they offer a place where people can go for consolation, inspiration, and direction on their path to mental health.

Identifying symptoms of worry and stress

Stress and anxiety can subtly permeate our everyday lives given the fast-paced nature of modern life. Encouraging mental well-being requires recognizing the early indicators of these emotional difficulties. We'll illuminate the subtle cues that indicate tension and anxiety in this inquiry, giving you the tools to successfully negotiate the complex emotional terrain.

1. Physical clues:Tense shoulders and neck muscles in particular.

* Recurrent migraines or headaches.

* Disrupted sleep patterns, such as excessive or insomniac sleep.

2. Emotional Changes:Enhanced irritation or fluctuations in mood.

* Extended periods of anxiety or fear.

* Having trouble focusing or choosing what to do.

3. Modifications in Behavior:Social disengagement or avoiding routine activities.

* Variations in appetite, such as overeating or undereating.

 * An increase in coping mechanisms such as alcohol or tobacco use.

Cognitive patterns include racing thoughts and persistent worry.

 * Enhanced negative self-talk and self-criticism.

 * Having trouble calming down or getting enough sleep.

5. Effect on Physical Health: * Weakened immune system, which makes infections more common.

 * Problems with the digestive system, such as IBS or stomachaches.

 * A worsening of pre-existing medical issues.

The sixth type of sleep disturbance is * Having trouble falling or staying asleep.

* Severe nightmares or insomnia.

* Feeling worn out even after getting enough sleep.

7. Modifications in Social Conduct: * Enhanced seclusion or evasion of social engagements.

* Tense friendships, family, or work ties.

* Having trouble connecting with others or expressing feelings.

8. Physical symptoms include: * Heart palpitations or an elevated heart rate; * Breathing difficulties or shallow breathing; * Dizziness or lightheadedness.

It's like reading the emotional weather report when you recognize these indicators; it gets you ready to react thoughtfully and carefully. When stress and anxiety are not managed, they can have an adverse effect on many aspects of life, including mental and physical health.

Chapter 6

Family-friendly First Aid

Life is unpredictable, and minor mishaps can happen at any moment. Chapter 6 is your family's guide to mastering the basics of first aid—an essential skillset that empowers you to respond confidently and effectively in times of need. Let's embark on this journey to create a safe haven for your loved ones, equipped with the knowledge to handle common injuries and emergencies.

1. Understanding the Basics:

* Remedy: Learn the fundamentals of first aid—knowing how to assess a situation and provide initial care.

* Explanation: Familiarize yourself with the ABCs of first aid: Airway, Breathing, and Circulation. Knowing when to call for professional help and how to perform basic life support can make a significant difference in critical situations.

2. Cuts and Scrapes:

* Remedy: Clean the wound with mild soap and water, apply an antiseptic ointment, and cover it with a sterile bandage.

*Explanation: Swift and proper care for cuts and scrapes helps prevent infections. Knowing how to clean and dress a wound ensures a quick and safe recovery.

3. Burns and Scalds:

* Remedy:Cool the burn with cold running water for at least 10 minutes and cover it with a clean, non-stick dressing.

* Explanation: Immediate cooling of burns helps alleviate pain and minimize damage. Avoid using ice directly on the burn, as it can worsen the injury.

4. Sprains and Strains:

* Remedy: Rest, ice, compression, and elevation (R.I.C.E.).

* Explanation: This classic formula for treating sprains and strains can significantly reduce swelling and promote healing. Knowing how to apply each element of R.I.C.E. is crucial for effective care.

5. Choking:

* Remedy: Perform the Heimlich maneuver for conscious choking victims or CPR for unconscious victims.

* Explanation: Being prepared to handle choking incidents, especially with young children, can be life-saving. Understanding the appropriate response based on the victim's condition is key.

6. Fractures and Dislocations:**

   * Remedy: Immobilize the injured area and seek professional medical help.

   * Explanation: Knowing how to provide initial support for fractures and dislocations minimizes further damage. Avoid moving the injured limb and stabilize it until professional medical assistance is available.

*7. Allergic Reactions:

   * Remedy: Administer an epinephrine auto-injector (if available) and seek emergency medical attention.

   * Explanation: Recognizing signs of severe allergic reactions, such as

anaphylaxis, and knowing how to use an auto-injector can be life-saving in critical situations.

8. Creating a Family First Aid Kit:

* Remedy: Assemble a first aid kit with essential supplies.

* Explanation: Prepare for emergencies by having a well-equipped first aid kit at home. Include items like bandages, antiseptic wipes, pain relievers, and emergency contact information.

Mastering family-friendly first aid is not about becoming a medical expert; it's about instilling confidence and preparedness within your family. By delving into the contents of this chapter, you're taking proactive steps to create a safer environment for your loved ones, turning your home into a haven of care and support. Remember, being prepared is not just a skill; it's an act of love for your family's well-being.

Creating a family first aid kits

creating a Family First Aid Kit: Your Essential Guide

A well-prepared family is a resilient family, and at the heart of that preparedness lies a thoughtfully assembled first aid kit. In times of minor mishaps or unforeseen emergencies, having the right supplies on hand can make a significant difference. This comprehensive guide walks you through the process of creating a family first aid kit, ensuring you're equipped to handle a variety of situations with confidence.

1. Selecting the Right Container:

   * Consideration:Choose a durable and portable container.

   * Explanation:Opt for a container that is sturdy, waterproof, and easily transportable. A plastic or metal box with compartments can help keep supplies organized.

2. Basic First Aid Supplies:

Essentials:

- Adhesive bandages in various sizes.

- Sterile gauze pads and adhesive tape.

- Antiseptic wipes or solution for cleaning wounds.

- Scissors and tweezers.

- Disposable gloves.

3 Medications:

Essentials:

- Pain relievers (acetaminophen, ibuprofen).

- Antihistamines for allergic reactions.

- Aspirin (for adults, if recommended by a healthcare provider).

4. Emergency Tools:

Essentials:

- Digital thermometer.

- Tweezers for splinter removal.

- Small flashlight with extra batteries.

- Safety pins.

5. Wound Care:

Essentials:

- Sterile saline solution for cleaning wounds.

- Hydrocortisone cream for itch relief.

- Burn ointment.

- Instant cold packs.

6. Respiratory Aids:

Essentials:

- Breathing barrier mask for CPR.

- Inhaler (if someone in the family has asthma).

- Antihistamine for allergic reactions involving respiratory symptoms.

7. Personal Items:

Essentials:

- Emergency contact list.

- List of allergies and medications for each family member.

- Personal hygiene items (hand sanitizer, tissues).

8. Additional Items for Specific Needs:

Considerations:

- EpiPen for severe allergic reactions (if prescribed).

- Medical information cards for chronic conditions.

- Specialized items for infants, elderly family members, or those with specific health needs.

9. First Aid Manual:

Consideration: Include a first aid manual or reference guide.

Explanation:Having a manual can guide you through basic first aid procedures and refresh your memory on proper techniques.

10. Regular Check and Replenishment:

* **Consideration:** Schedule routine checks and replenish supplies.

* **Explanation:** Ensure that your first aid kit remains up-to-date. Check expiration dates on medications and replace any used or expired items promptly.

.

Chapter 7

Women's and Men's Health

It is essential to comprehend the distinct features of men's and women's health in order to promote general wellbeing. Insights, preventative strategies, and useful advice for leading a healthy and balanced life are provided in Chapter 7, which explores the unique factors that influence the health of men and women.

1. Essentials of Women's Health: Managing the Lifecycle

Examine the fundamentals of reproductive health, including family planning and menstrual cycles. Recognize typical worries and discover the significance of routine gynecological exams.

* Pregnancy and Motherhood: Learn about the nuances of becoming pregnant, giving birth, and caring for yourself thereafter. Explore the mental and physical facets of becoming a mother and learn how to have a safe pregnancy.

2. Men's Health Fundamentals: Looking Past the Surface*m * **Proactive Wellness: Talk about the importance of men's preventative health practices. Enable men to take control of their health

by providing them with regular checkups and information on risk factors for diseases including prostate health and cardiovascular disease.

* Mental Health: Dispel the myth that men's mental health is inferior. Examine methods for reducing stress, taking care of mental health issues, and promoting emotional health.

3. Common Health Issues to Be Aware of:

* Cardiovascular Health: Learn how crucial heart health is for both sexes. Talk about lifestyle decisions including a balanced diet and frequent exercise that support cardiovascular health.

* Nutrition and Fitness: Learn about gender-specific fitness regimens and dietary advice. Stress the importance of physical activity and a balanced diet in preserving good health.

4. Hormonal Health: Equilibrium Management for Both Sexes

* Women's Hormonal Health: Recognize the hormonal shifts that occur in women at various phases of life, including puberty and menopause. Talk about common issues including hormone imbalances and how they affect general health. Men's Hormonal Health: Examine how hormones, particularly testosterone levels

and aging, affect men's health. Talk about the importance of hormonal balance and possible remedies.

5. Mental and Emotional Health: Closing the Gender Divide

* Women's Emotional Health: Provided insight into the particular emotional difficulties that women may encounter, such as mood disorders and the effects of hormone changes. Talk about coping strategies and getting help. guys's Emotional Health: Talking to guys about mental health should no longer be stigmatized. Examine cultural norms and

offer advice on how to deal with stress, anxiety, and depression.

6. Intimacy and Sexual Health: A Holistic View

* Women's Sexual Health: Talk about how important it is for women to have good sexual health, including how to use contraception and maintain good reproductive and sexual health. Promote awareness and honest dialogue.

* **Men's Sexual Health:** Examine the variables that impact men's sexual health, such as prostate health and erectile dysfunction. Stress the importance of routine examinations and discussion with

medical professionals.7. Growing Old With Grace: An Throughout Life PathThe Aging of Women: ** Talk about how women should age, including hormone fluctuations, bone health, and ways to stay active. Examine the ideas of proactive health management and graceful aging.

* The Aging of Men: Talk about common health issues that affect men as they age, such as cardiovascular changes, prostate health, and preserving mental clarity. Stress the value of routine health screenings.

Chapter 8

Navigating the Healthcare System

Being able to navigate the healthcare system is a critical ability that allows people to obtain and benefit from the best care available. Insights, advice, and useful tactics are provided in Chapter 8 to help you navigate the complexities of the healthcare system and make an informed and easy journey through it.

1. Understanding Healthcare Basics: Health Insurance Overview: Learn about the fundamentals of health insurance, such

as coverage options, policy types, and jargon.

- Primary Care Physicians:Acknowledge the importance of primary care physicians in the management of general health.

2. Putting Together a Healthcare Team:

- Selecting Healthcare Providers:Discover how to choose specialists, general practitioners, and other medical experts in accordance with patient needs.

Patient Advocacy:Recognize the significance of standing up for your rights and demands in terms of healthcare

.3. Getting Around Health Insurance: - Knowing Your Plan:Examine the various parts of health insurance policies, such as co-payments, deductibles, premiums, and coverage limitations.

- Using Preventive Services: Examine the benefits of insurance-covered preventive services and their part in preserving health.

4. Making Informed Healthcare Decisions:

- Informed Consent:Recognize the significance of actively engaging in healthcare decision-making and the idea of informed consent.

Researching Treatment Options:Develop your ability to investigate and assess available treatments, getting second opinions as needed.

5.Managing Healthcare Costs: - Budgeting for Healthcare: Create plans for comprehending medical bills and negotiating prices, among other things, in order to budget for and manage healthcare costs.

Prescription Medication Costs: Examine your choices, including patient assistance programs and generic substitutes, for controlling the expense of prescription medications.

6. Electronic Health Records (EHRs): - Knowing EHRs: Acquire knowledge of

the advantages, accessibility, and significance of maintaining the security of personal health information.

Managing Personal Health Data:Examine methods and resources for keeping a health history and other personal health information.

7. Managing Specialty Care: - Referrals and Specialist Appointments:Recognize how to get specialist appointments organized and how to get referrals for specialty care.

Working with Specialists:Examine efficient methods for communicating health issues and working with specialists.

8. Emergencies and Immediate Care:
Recognizing the Difference Between Emergency and Urgent Care:Find out when to seek each type of care as well as how to discern between emergencies and urgent care scenarios.

Developing Emergency Plans: Make emergency plans, which should include having a list of emergency contacts and being aware of the closest emergency facilities.9. Telehealth Services:
Exploring Telehealth:Recognize the advantages of telehealth services, such as

remote monitoring and virtual consultations.

Getting Ready for Telehealth Appointments: Discover how to get ready for and maximize telehealth appointments so that you can communicate with medical professionals efficiently.

10. Patient Rights and Responsibilities: - Knowing Your Rights: Educate yourself on patient rights, such as the right to medical record access, informed consent, and confidentiality.

Taking Responsibility: Recognize that patients have a responsibility to participate actively in their healthcare, including giving accurate medical histories and adhering to recommended treatment regimens.

It takes a team effort from patients, healthcare providers, and support systems to navigate the healthcare system. Chapter 8 gives you the information and resources you need to successfully negotiate the healthcare system's intricacies and promotes an informed and proactive approach to personal well-being.

Comprehending medical visits and examinations

Maintaining good health requires understanding and utilizing doctor visits and check-ups to the fullest. Here's a guide to help you make the most of these appointments:

1. Making an Appointment-Frequent Exams:Consider your age, gender, and any underlying medical concerns when scheduling regular check-ups. These could be gynecological examinations, yearly physicals, or targeted testing.

Urgent Needs:Make an appointment as soon as possible with your healthcare practitioner if you have any urgent health issues.

2. Getting Ready for the Visit: - Medical History:Gather a thorough medical history

that includes previous surgeries, prescription drugs currently being taken, and any known allergies.

List of Concerns: Make a list of any particular health issues or inquiries you would like to bring up during the appointment.

3. Information about Insurance and Administration:InsuranceDetails:Please bring your insurance card and any other required documentation.

Payment and Co-payments:Recognize your insurance coverage, comply with any co-payment requirements, and be ready to make any necessary payments.

4. Check-In and Arrival:Get there early: To ensure a seamless check-in procedure and to finish any paperwork, try to come a bit early.

Update Information:Notify the receptionist of any modifications to your insurance details or contact information.

5.ThroughourtheVisitHonestCommunicati on:Communicate honestly and openly with your healthcare practitioner. Please share any symptoms, health changes, or worries you may have.

*Ask Inquiries:** Never be afraid to ask questions concerning your condition, available treatments, or any medical guidance you may get.

**6. Physical Exams: **- **Standard Exams: ** Anticipate regular physical checkups, which can involve monitoring your weight, heart rate, blood pressure, and other critical indicators.

Traditional Tests: It may be advised to undergo specialized tests or screenings based on your age, gender, and medical history.

7. Laboratory Examinations and Screenings: - **Hematological

Testing:** To check on things like blood sugar, cholesterol, or organ function, your doctor might prescribe blood tests.

Imaging Research: Your doctor may suggest imaging tests like MRIs or X-rays if necessary.

8. Immunizations and Preventive Measures: - **Vaccinations:** Keep your immunizations current, particularly those that are advised for your age group and medical conditions.

- **preventative Advice:** Pay attention to what your healthcare provider advises regarding lifestyle modifications, health screenings, and preventative actions.

9. Follow-Up Plans: - **Medication Adjustments:** Know when and how to take any recommended drugs. Talk about any possible adverse effects.

   - **Repeated Schedules:** As directed by your physician, make any necessary follow-up appointments or screenings.

10. Post-Visit Reflection: - **Review Recommendations:** Give careful consideration to any advice or guidelines that your healthcare practitioner has given you.

   - **Medication Adherence:** Comply with treatment programs and prescription drugs as directed.

11. Electronic Records and Patient Portals: - **Getting Information:** Learn how to use patient portals, also known as electronic health records, to speak with your healthcare physician and view test results and appointment history.

12. Seeking Second Opinions: - **Thought:** Do not be afraid to consult with a different healthcare provider for a second opinion if you are dealing with a complicated medical matter.

Recall that the most important things in healthcare are proactive involvement and good communication. Frequent check-ups offer the chance for early health issue detection, preventive care, and building a cooperative relationship with your healthcare provider

Conclusion

: Final Thoughts and Motivation

As we come to the end of this investigation into family health and healthcare, it is evident that information, proactive decision-making, and supportive communities are the many threads that make up our complex web of wellbeing. Adopting a holistic approach that takes into account not only the health of the individual but also the interrelated dynamics within families is crucial as we negotiate the intricacies of healthcare.

*Concluding Remarks: * Every stride made in the direction of family health education, prevention, and well-informed decision-making enhances the resiliency and vitality of the family as a whole. Keep in mind that maintaining good health is a journey, and that little actions over time can frequently add up to big gains.

Encouragement: I would want to urge you to embark on your health journey with an attitude of empowerment and curiosity. Assume responsibility for your health, communicate honestly with medical staff, and instill a healthy lifestyle in your family. Little adjustments can have profound effects, and every wise decision spreads wellbeing across the community.

Sources for Additional Assistance:
Investigate reliable sources and groups committed to advancing health and wellbeing for continuing assistance and comprehensive information on family health and medical care:

1. The **[Centers for Disease Control and Prevention (CDC)](https://www.cdc.gov/):** An extensive source of knowledge on a variety of health-related subjects,

preventative measures, and public health campaigns.

2.   **[Mayo Clinic](https://www.mayoclinic.org/):** A reliable resource for medical information, including advice on lifestyle choices, therapies, and insights into a range of health issues.

3. The American Academy of Family Physicians'   site **[FamilyDoctor.org](https://familydoctor.org/):**   offers   details   on   patient education, family health, and wellness.

The National Institute of Child Health and Human   Development   (NICHD)   is   a non-profit organization that focuses on improving maternal and child health and well-being throughout life.

5. **[American Heart Association](https://www.heart.org/):** A great source of information about cardiovascular health, including advice on leading a heart-healthy lifestyle and preventing illness.

Recall that asking for help and information is not a sign of weakness, but rather of power. Make use of these resources to broaden your horizons, take control of your decisions, and improve your family's quality of life.

Every person and family has a distinct tale to share in the fabric of health. I hope your path is one of resiliency, vigor, and the community acceptance of wellbeing.

Review Page

Dear Readers

I hope you are well-versed on (family health and medical guide) as I write this message. Your opinions about the book are really valuable to me as the author.

I would appreciate it if you would consider giving a review of [family health and medical guide] if you have enjoyed reading it. In addition to offering insightful criticism, your review will encourage other readers to pick up the book.

I would be grateful for your honest evaluation, and I look forward to hearing your point of view.

I appreciate your participation in this literary journey and eagerly await your assessment.

Warm Regards

(Florence J. Jacoby]

[Author of "family health and medical guide"]

www.ingramcontent.com/pod-product-compliance
Lightning Source LLC
Chambersburg PA
CBHW070847260726
48661CB00004B/1279